# FILL THE GEL BOTTLES

# FILL THE GEL BOTTLES

A STUDENT'S GUIDE TO SUCCESS IN SCHOOL AND BEYOND

BY RONALD EUSTIS

**Ronald Eustis**
**Fill The Gel Bottles**



Published by Spines

ISBN: 979-8-89569-295-0

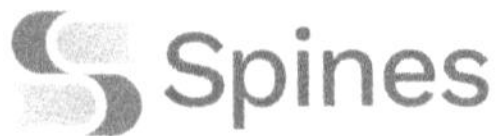

# CONTENTS

•

If you want to stand out……
FILL THE GEL BOTTLES

If you want to succeed……
FILL THE GEL BOTTLES

If you want to get hired……
FILL THE GEL BOTTLES

BY RONALD EUSTIS
(RVT, RDCS)

# THE END

"IT'S THE END, NOW LET'S BEGIN"
-RONALD EUSTIS

Hello, fellow world of ultrasound knowledge seekers. Are you ready to embark on a journey into the wild world of Ultrasound Tech? Welcome to "Fill the Gel Bottles: A Student's Guide to Success"—the book that hopes to make you laugh a little, make you wonder what the hell have I got myself into a little, and hopefully help you make your first step out of the classroom and into the real world a good one.

You may think, "What in the world is so important about filling gel bottles?" Well, let me be the first to tell you it's all about filling the gel bottles. If you can confidently and expertly fill the gel bottles in your school's lab, a clinic, or wherever you end up, you will have completed one task. Although it may be easy, it will send you in the right direction for the day, completing one task after another. At the end of the day, especially a tough day, you'll at least be able to say, "Well, at least I filled the gel bottles." What you're about to read will be something other than some boring advice or an ordinary old guide. No, no, no! This guide will help you turn your ultrasound fantasy into a real-life adventure.

Who will hire someone with little skill, some basic knowledge, and no experience? That's the million-dollar question. It's more like the 74,000-dollar question. It's not medical school, after all. The problem is that they expect you to know as much as an MD from day one in the disease-ridden, pathology-rich real world. It's only life and death we're talking about here. Okay, not always, but sometimes.

So, whether you're a frightened ultrasound rookie in your first class or a confident senior who can see that externship light at the end of the tunnel, "Fill the Gel Bottles" is the book for you. Why fill the gel bottles? Only because it's the easiest, most important thing you will ever do, and throughout this guide, you will find out why. This book will guide you through the struggles you will face as you enter the exciting world of Ultrasound Tech with some humor, experience-based advice, and stories to help prepare you for this journey.

If you're ready, grab your gel bottles, put on your lab coat, and wait a second; you don't need those for this. Grab a snack and your reading glasses if needed, and find a quiet place to dive headfirst into the dark, deep waters of the beautiful world of ultrasound.

# A BRIEF HISTORY

"IT'S WHAT YOU LEARN AFTER YOU KNOW IT ALL THAT COUNTS."
-JOHN WOODEN

Once upon a time, a scientist discovered the magic of ultrasound in a galaxy far, far away. It was this galaxy, but you get the idea. Let's briefly dive into the history of ultrasound. This mysterious technology has changed how we see and understand the human body. Long ago, but not that long, some brilliant minds began the epic pursuit of understanding the character of sound and its interaction with matter.

Pierre Curie is the brilliant scientist who first discovered the piezoelectric effect, a phenomenon where certain crystals would produce an electrical charge when subjected to mechanical pressure. Little did Curie know that his discovery would lay the foundation for the power of ultrasound. Inspired by Curie's work, scientists embarked on a journey to harness the power of sound waves. Transducers were designed, which consisted of piezoelectric crystals that could emit and receive sound waves. Transducers have become the sonographer's magic wand and the heart of the ultrasound field.

You'll find ultrasound is an art as you master the wielding of sound waves and unlock the skills needed to control the transducer. The power is in creating an echoing sound and vibration masterpiece within the human body. When the sound creates waves and enters the body, they encounter different tissues, allowing harmonious echoes to return and beautiful images to be produced.

If the transducer is the heart of ultrasound, the machine is the soul. The gel is the crucial component that serves as a coupling agent, which forms a vital continuous connection, enabling the effortless transfer of energy through the body for accurate imaging. Scientists could interpret these echoes through the machine, transforming them into recognizable images. Physicians could now quickly peek into the human body. They began using this noninvasive, painless tool. It allowed them to glance into the inner realm of the body, helping them to provide treatment to their patients more quickly and efficiently.

Ultrasound and the ultrasound tech were born. The machine and the tech have become essential medical tools, aiding in diagnosing ailments and monitoring patients' health, from unborn children to our senior citizens. So began the vital habit of "filling the gel bottles" and the ultrasound tech's never-ending search for the perfect image.

As time and technology progressed, specialized transducers were created, which could explore further and deeper into the body, expanding the field and building new roads of possibility. Veins, arteries, abdominal organs, the heart, and the brain were now visualized through ultrasound. Soon after, a powerful collaboration with X-ray, MRI, and CT scans began creating a comprehensive portrait of the body. This dynamic collaboration of sound waves, x-rays, and magnetic fields allowed doctors to view the body from multiple angles, lighting the way to less invasive diagnostics. The scientific journey continues today and promises to surge forward as we head into our limitless future.

## BE CURIOUS

"CURIOSITY DID NOT KILL THE CAT."
-RONALD EUSTIS

"Curiosity killed the cat" is a proverb that warns about the dangers of being too curious or nosy. This well-known saying suggests excessive curiosity may lead to trouble and unintended consequences. Curiosity itself is not the problem. It's about how curiosity is expressed. Curiosity is a valuable trait that can lead to personal growth, learning, and positive experiences. On occasion, curiosity may lead to unexpected outcomes, like the unfortunate demise of a cat, but do not worry; they have nine lives. For instance, you may be curious if you can use a microwave to warm the gel in a bottle after filling it. The answer is yes, but I will leave it up to you to discover how long to leave the gel bottle in the microwave before it explodes.

Natural curiosity can benefit you by enriching your personal, professional, and intellectual experiences. Maybe you're still curious why it's crucial to "fill the gel bottles" each morning. Hopefully, the answer will be apparent to you soon. Curiosity can drive you to move forward and seek answers. As you enter the field, timely expression of interest is vital.

Imagine the tech you are shadowing in your externship is spending an unusual amount of time capturing images of a particular piece of anatomy. You know the protocol; the tech takes many more pictures than usual. You have not noted any apparent pathology. Is this the time to let your curiosity run wild and ask them why they are taking extra images? If you said no, you are correct. This is the most essential time to be quiet. Sometimes, curiosity and excitement can get the best of us. This experienced tech is hard at work and needs to concentrate. Now is not the time to ask questions because you don't want to alarm the patient or distract the tech. You may think you're asking a simple question about ultrasound, but it may make the patient feel uncomfortable, nervous, or worried. Please make a note of it. Review the study and the preliminary findings with the tech in the hallway or office. They will appreciate your silence and the fact that you're curious and there to learn.

Here are some ways in which curiosity can be advantageous:

**Continuous Learning**: Curiosity fuels a desire to learn.

**Problem-Solving**: Curious individuals are more willing to explore various solutions and perspectives, which can lead to improved problem-solving and creative thinking.

**Adaptability:** Curiosity helps you adapt more quickly to new situations and environments. You're more likely to embrace change and look for opportunities within it rather than resisting or fearing it.

**Critical Thinking**: Curiosity encourages you to question

assumptions, analyze information, and evaluate different viewpoints.

**Increased Empathy**: Curiosity about other people's experiences, cultures, and perspectives fosters empathy.

**Professional Growth**: Curious individuals are often more adaptable in the workplace, likely to seek new skills and take on challenging projects.

**Brain Health**: A curious mind is more active and engaged.

**Enhanced Creativity**: Curious minds tend to connect seemingly unrelated ideas, leading to alternative solutions.

**Open-Mindedness**: Curiosity encourages open-mindedness and a willingness to consider different perspectives.

**Increased Confidence**: You will accumulate knowledge and skills through your curiosity-driven pursuits, giving you confidence.

Cultivating curiosity involves embracing a mindset of exploration, asking questions, and being open to change. Incorporating curiosity into your life consists of maintaining an open attitude, embracing uncertainty, and actively seeking opportunities for learning and exploration. If you're willing to stay curious, it will unlock numerous opportunities and give you the knowledge and confidence to take advantage of them as they arise.

## BE FEARLESS

"THERE IS NOTHING TO FEAR
BUT FEAR ITSELF."
-FRANKLIN D. ROOSEVELT

You will feel many emotions when you get out in the field. Excited one moment, anxious the next, nervous, happy, or who knows what. The one emotion you will feel but must not let rule is fear. You must be brave and have the courage to dive in head first. Hospitals can be frightening places with sick people, overworked nurses, and scary doctors. Don't let fear take over. Be prepared for anything and go for it. The act of filling the gel bottles can be grounding. It's a time when you are in control and can take a deep breath before heading out to do a study, which is creating some fear or anxiety. A great thing about ultrasound gel is that it has never hurt anybody. Sure, it may be cold, which will get you an ear full of complaints, but there is no actual harm being done. If I had a dime for the number of times I added gel when it was unnecessary, I'd have a lot of dimes. In those stressful moments when you can't find the anatomy or can't quite get the image you're looking for, applying more gel and taking a deep breath comes in handy. In other words, another good reason to keep the gel bottles full is for your mental health.

I recall a day early in my externship when the tech I was shadowing and I walked into a patient's room. The patient weighed about 400 Lbs. We were there to do a venous study to rule out a DVT. I set up the machine and prepped the patient. We look at the patient, and there is no groin in sight. The tech looks at the patient, pauses, then turns to me and hands me the probe. She says, "Okay, go for it." I did not hesitate. I grabbed the ultrasound probe and boldly went where I hoped the groin would be. I had to go in under the belly fat about as far as my elbow, but I found the Common Femoral Vein and continued the study the best I could from there. I believe this was a test of sorts. Although the tech wasn't super excited to do this study, she certainly could have. She wanted to see what I was made of. After that, she was always happy to have me shadow her and have me do her dirty work. The best part is how eager she was to tell all the other techs of my triumph. My fearless reputation was established. He will "fill the gel bottles," and he's willing to do what it takes to get the job done.

Fear is natural. Unfortunately, fear can also become a limiting factor, holding us back from pursuing our dreams and getting things done. Anxiety and stress can be turned into a positive force driving us forward. You may have learned by now that embracing your fears is the first step towards conquering them. Rather than avoiding situations that make you anxious, face them willingly. I knew I always wanted to work in a private practice. I was fearful of hospitals and felt nervous in that environment. I also learned that having ultrasound experience in a hospital would set me up for more tremendous success. I chose to take an externship in a hospital environment. This exposure helped to desensitize my mind and reduced the fear and anxiety over time. I was exposed quickly to various pathologies, allowing me to gain real-world experience.

Self-talk can help you rationalize your fear. Ask yourself: What is the worst that could happen? Usually, our fears will be magnified by our imagination. By confronting them with logic, you can diminish their power. Try to view fear as a challenge to overcome rather than an obstacle. Significant achievements require individuals to step out of their comfort zones. Embracing fear as a necessary part of growth can empower you to take bolder steps.

We are all going to make mistakes as we go along. Learning from those mistakes is what helps us grow into experienced ultrasound professionals. Surround yourself with a supportive network of friends, family, mentors, and fellow students. Sharing your fears and receiving encouragement from others can bolster your confidence and provide you with valuable perspectives.

Ultimately, the most effective way to become fearless is to take action. Act despite your fear. You'll build resilience and courage as you overcome discomfort and face your fears head-on. Fear has a way of losing its grip when you confront it directly. Being fearless is not the absence of fear; it's the mastery of it. By embracing your fears and shifting your perspective, you can transform uncomfortable or scary situations into empowering ones.

# BE FLEXIBLE

"YOU'RE JUST STANDING THERE;
MIGHT AS WELL STRETCH,"
-RONALD EUSTIS

As an ultrasound tech, you better be flexible. I don't just mean having a flexible schedule or mindset. I mean this in a truly physical sense. If you have yet to figure it out, this career is an athletic endeavor in many ways. Whether you work in a clinic or a hospital, you will soon find out it requires some strength, some stamina, some balance, and most definitely some flexibility. Proper body mechanics and physical health will go a long way in keeping you healthy and fit in this career.

If you work in a hospital, you must move that ultrasound machine down long hallways, into crowded elevators, and often into tight rooms. Once in the room, you may have to move furniture and help the patient get into position for the study. It's best to return everything just how you found it; otherwise, you may have one of those hangry nurses after you. If you work in a clinic, you'll set up the room, walk back and forth, get the patients from the waiting room, and clean the room after each study. We still need to discuss the part where you're doing the ultrasound. Even under the perfect conditions, performing hours of ultrasound can tax your back, neck, wrists, and shoulders.

News flash: Conditions allowing for proper body mechanics and movement could be better in most clinical and hospital settings. As far as strength and stamina go, you can stay in shape just by going to work. I recall times in the hospital when I would get 20-25,000 steps in daily. Using good body mechanics and asking for help when needed covers the strength department for the most part. The critical component to maintain is flexibility.

Stretching is often underestimated yet pivotal in daily movement. It's not just about touching your toes or bending like a gymnast; stretching is a cornerstone of overall health and fitness. As you may know, our bodies comprise complex, interconnected networks of tissues, muscles, and joints. This finely tuned machine requires lubrication to function smoothly. Stretching creates the oil that keeps your physiological machinery running at its best.

Joints act as the hinges between bones, enabling movement and flexibility. Regular stretching promotes the circulation of synovial fluid, nourishing and lubricating the joints, thus reducing the risk of injuries and maintaining longevity.

As stated earlier, your day at work is an active one. Stretching works as a warm-up and or cool-down ritual for muscles. Before work, dynamic stretching readies muscles for action by increasing blood flow and oxygen supply. After work, static stretching can help in muscle recovery by alleviating tension and preventing post-activity soreness. It's like a therapeutic massage that your muscles give themselves.

Ultrasound often involves prolonged sitting, standing, and hunching over the machine or patient. Poor posture can lead to muscular imbalances. Regular stretching helps correct imbalances by elongating tight muscles and strengthening weak ones, improving posture, better balance, and reducing strain on your spine.

Physical and mental well-being are intricately connected. The tension held in your muscles can mirror the stress in your mind. Stretching provides a two-fold benefit—stretching releases muscular tension, contributing to a relaxed feeling. Second, stretching can be a mindfulness exercise, offering a mental break from the chaos of daily life. Consider your muscles and tendons as rubber bands. Stretching these "bands" regularly increases their flexibility and resilience. So, when sudden movements or stresses occur, your body is less likely to incur strains, sprains, or tears. Incorporating proper stretching into your routine is a preemptive measure against potential injuries.

Do you know where the true beauty in stretching lies? You don't need specialized equipment or a gym membership to practice. You will have times when you are busy and other times when you are not. For instance, you rush to a patient's room for a study, but the patient has undergone X-rays. The nurse says they will be back "shortly." There's not enough time to see another patient. Downtime is a perfect time to do some stretches. There will be many opportunities like this throughout the day. "You're just standing there; might as well stretch." A few minutes here and there throughout the day can make a difference. Here are some tips to make stretching a consistent part of your routine:

**Dynamic Warm-up**: Incorporate dynamic stretches before work to prime your muscles for activity.

**Static Stretching**: After work, spend a few minutes performing static stretches for the major muscle groups.

**Mindful Moments**: Integrate brief stretching breaks throughout your day to combat the effects of prolonged sitting, standing, and mental fatigue.

**Yoga and Pilates**: Consider participating in yoga or Pilates classes to combine stretching with mindful movement.

Stretching is a soft yet powerful note that harmonizes the body and mind. Embrace its simplicity, and you'll find yourself reaping the rewards of increased flexibility, reduced stress, and enhanced well-being. If you create the habit of stretching, your body will thank you for years to come.

# HABITS

"WE ARE WHAT WE REPEATEDLY DO. EXCELLENCE, THEN, IS NOT AN ACT BUT A HABIT."

-WILL DURANT

Do you have any habits? We all have habits, some good and some bad ones. Believe it or not, the rhythm of life is often dictated by our habits. You know, those subconscious routines that guide our actions and decisions throughout the day. Habits shape our lives profoundly, from when we wake up in the morning to when we go to bed at night. We can tilt the scale when we consciously design these habits to work in our favor. The concept of habits and its smaller counterpart, micro-habits, is a powerful tool for personal growth, productivity, and overall well-being.

The definition of a habit is a regular tendency or practice, especially one that is hard to give up. If we create good habits, like "filling the gel bottles," they are just as hard to give up as the bad ones. We can use this to our advantage. For example, it will become effortless if you create the habit of showing up early. The art of the micro-habits falls into two categories. The first is when we tie a small habit onto a bigger one. For example, once you create the habit of showing up early to work, it will signal you and give you the time to make smaller habits like filling the gel bottles and ensuring things are ready for the day. This will set you up for success and show your employer or potential employer who you are and what they can expect if they hire you. The other type of micro-habit is beneficial when trying to create larger ones. You want to make a habit of keeping your workspace tidy. Pick one small thing, like always re-stocking your towels at the end of the day. Once you re-stock the towels, it leads you to tidy the rest of the space because your energy and focus have led you there.

Every habit has a ripple effect that extends far beyond its immediate action. Simple daily routines compound over time, creating profound behavior, mindset, and accomplishments. Have you heard of the "habit loop?" It's a three-step process that explains how habits are formed and sustained: cue, routine, and reward. The queue acts as a trigger, signaling the brain to initiate a practice. It could be anything from a specific time of day to the start of an ultrasound protocol. The routine is, for example, the protocol; the cue prompts the action. Finally, the reward is a positive outcome, reinforcing the habit loop. The goal of an ultrasound protocol is to capture all the necessary images. When you nail your protocols, it signals to the ordering physician and the Lead Technician in your department that you are a serious candidate.

Creating excellent workplace habits will make your daily routine go more smoothly. When something becomes a habit, you no longer have to put much thought into it. It's important to remember that habit formation is gradual, whether through traditional rituals or micro-habits. Instant transformation is rare, and setbacks are part of the experience. However, the consistent application of small actions can yield remarkable long-term results. Patience and self-compassion are crucial.

Habits are not a one-size-fits-all solution. What works for one person might not work for another, and experimentation is critical to finding the right approach. Like riding a bike, habits can become automatic. Intentionally creating positive habits can be powerful and give you an advantage in the field.

Habits and micro-habits can empower us to shape our lives intentionally. By understanding the habit loop and embracing the concept of micro-habits, we can harness their power to drive personal growth, cultivate positive behaviors, and lead to excellence. Remember, it's not the size of the habit that matters most but the consistent commitment to positive change.

# DON'T BE LATE

"DON'T WORRY ABOUT BEING LATE,
JUST BE EARLY."
-UNKNOWN

The advice from this quote is powerful, whether getting to the airport, arriving for an interview, or just getting to work. There is a power or magic to it. Have you ever been running late trying to catch a flight? Remember how many delays present themselves and how fast an hour can go by. On the other hand, when you arrive early, the lines seem shorter, and you ask yourself why you got to the airport so early. I don't know about you, but being chill waiting to get on the plane versus the stress of rushing through the airport hoping you'll catch that flight is like night and day.

There is the same energy when you arrive at work early. Things work out more smoothly. You may also find that people look at you and treat you differently when you're the one who is always early, as opposed to the person who is rushing and always running late. This is an excellent opportunity to fill the gel bottles. Arriving early and ensuring the gel bottles are full is critical to getting noticed at your externship or new job. Another more well-known cliché is "the early bird catches the worm." As an early bird myself, I can tell you that's true. I don't eat worms, but I love my coffee. What gets you going? When you get a head start on your daily tasks, you'll find more freedom to learn, listen, and grow.

One morning in my externship, after filling the gel bottles, I was moving the machine through the long hallways of the hospital when I got a call from the tech I was shadowing for the day. She asked me to set up the room for a carotid study. She said she was running late and to go ahead and start. (Get it?) When that call comes, I guarantee your heart will start pounding, and you'll get a pep in your step. You'll quickly go into protocol review mode. You'll probably get off the wrong floor and head in the wrong direction down the hallway. When you finally get there, though, you'll be ready.

I calmly introduced myself to the patient and informed them that their MD had requested an ultrasound of the Carotid artery in their neck. The other thing to consider when you get this call is that time is paramount. It is not because the physician needs this study right away. It's because the tech said you could get started. This means they are on their way. If you take too long to find the room, move all the furniture, and put information in the machine, you may have blown your chance. Once that tech arrives, it will be time to play a familiar game called Pass the Probe. Don't think for one second; they will sit there and look over your shoulder while you, the student, try to visualize the PROX RT CCA. Here it goes. I placed the probe on the patient's neck in the correct location, with the notch facing the right way. It looked calcified on the grayscale, much more than my fellow healthy young classmates.

You say to yourself, okay, I still have time. I turn on it like a pro, get that nice sagittal view, throw on the color box, and nothing, no flow. Without experience, your first impression is that you're doing wrong. Is my scale too high? Is the color box at the proper angle? Do I have enough gel? Unfortunately, this feeling stays with you until you gain the necessary experience and confidence. It takes a while. As it turns out, the patient's Carotid artery was completely occluded. When the tech arrived to take over shortly after, she was all business, “Let me see that probe.” I was early, and I had gained the tech’s trust. I was rewarded with an opportunity.

At last, disease! I can still clearly see that occluded Carotid artery. That's the good news: once you see stuff like this, you always remember it, and it helps you build your arsenal of experience, which will guide you in the future. These critical experiences are granted to those who arrive early, stay late, and fill the gel bottles.

The takeaway is that being early and filling the gel bottles is about something other than being on time. It's all part of setting yourself up for success. It lends itself to favorable judgment about your character, ambition, and work ethic. The Lead Tech can be late every morning, but it will count against you if you are even late once, at least in the crucial externship phase and early career days.

## JANE AND JOHNNY

"ANTICIPATE PEOPLE'S NEEDS,
AND YOU WILL MAKE YOURSELF A
VALUABLE ASSET."
-RONALD EUSTIS

Have you ever been in a situation where the person you're with seems to anticipate your every need? Maybe it was your mom or dad standing in the doorway with the sweater you forgot as you returned to get it. Have you ever climbed out of the pool and someone was standing there, ready to wrap a warm towel around you? What about the classmate who hands you a topped-off bottle of warm gel as you sit down to start a study? If so, you can appreciate this idea. You most likely were grateful for the person who was there for you and anticipated your needs. People love this. When you anticipate a person's needs, they see you as reliable, helpful, and compassionate. You become a Jane or Johnny on the spot; everybody wants to work with someone like that. A Johnny or Jane on the spot is the one who hands you a bottle of warm gel, a pen, a dry towel, or a helping hand when needed and without being asked.

Few skills are more impactful than anticipating another person's needs. This remarkable ability is a testament to our capacity for understanding, compassion, and proactive support. Whether among colleagues, patients, doctors, or the all-powerful nurse, the skill of foreseeing and fulfilling another's needs can enrich our interactions and foster deeper relationships. You can skillfully operate an incredibly sophisticated machine, but your ability to create meaningful relationships will allow you the opportunity to excel and enjoy being an ultrasound tech.

Doctors may be the key holders, but nurses are the gatekeepers. This is an important fact to remember. Nurses can make or break your day in many ways. Once you work in the field, being in the nurse's good graces is essential. You can do this by listening to their requests and consistently offering help. Showing up with chocolates or donuts never hurts. Doing little things for the department that are not specifically in your job description will be enough to set you apart. For example, remove and replace the dirty laundry or change the linen on a gurney to help the nurse prepare for the next patient. It will not go unnoticed, and it will be appreciated.

Anticipating people’s needs is a powerful way to strengthen the bonds between individuals. When we demonstrate that we genuinely care about another person's well-being and are attentive to their needs, it fosters a sense of trust and security. Understanding someone's unspoken desires can make them feel valued and appreciated. This will strengthen the emotional connection between them and the one who has anticipated their needs. As ultrasound techs, we are not just punching a clock. We are part of a team of healthcare providers working together for the greater good of each patient. When team members are attuned to each other's needs, they can collaboratively tackle challenges and support one another.

Anticipation of other's needs is an art. When we pay close attention to the subtle cues and signals others emit, we're better equipped to engage in meaningful conversations. In a professional setting, the ability to anticipate the needs of colleagues and teammates can significantly impact teamwork and productivity. These cues often reveal what someone may be hesitant or unable to express directly. By preemptively acknowledging and addressing these needs, we create an environment where people feel comfortable. When your patients are satisfied with you, it's a win. When your co-workers are comfortable with you, It's a win. When your employer is pleased with you, it's a win. This synergy leads to an enhanced, harmonious work environment. Trying to anticipate another person's needs often inspires them to do the same in return. This reciprocal behavior improves the overall quality of the relationship. If you're always the Jane or Johnny on the spot, especially during your externship, it will incentivize the tech you're shadowing to return the favor. In our case, the favor will be getting your hand on the probe and scanning in real-life situations.

The art of anticipating another person's needs goes beyond mind reading; it requires genuine care, attention, and active listening. By putting ourselves in the shoes of those around us, we can create an environment of empathy, trust, and confidence. As we cultivate this skill, we elevate our relationships to new heights, making our interactions more meaningful, fulfilling, and enduring. In a world where personal connections are cherished, the power of anticipation stands as a beacon of human connection. Why not strive to be a Jane or a Johnny on the spot?

# BUILD YOUR NETWORK

"EVERYONE SHOULD BUILD THEIR NETWORK BEFORE THEY NEED IT."
-DAVE DELANEY

In career development, networking is a crucial component of success. While it might seem like a buzzword or a practice reserved for professionals already engaging in business, the truth is that networking is an essential skill for anyone embarking on a new career. I am talking about the importance of relationship building. When you are in school, you can build substantial relationships with your fellow students and your professors. These are powerful relationships that can carry you into the future.

At its core, networking is about building and nurturing relationships that can support your professional journey. It's not just about building your Facebook, Instagram, and TikTok communities. Effective networking is about creating genuine, mutually beneficial relationships. It's an ongoing process that involves engaging with people, sharing information, and helping others in your network as much as you seek help.

I have an idea. Fill the gel bottles! One way to gain the appreciation of your fellow students and the respect of your lab instructor is to get in early and ensure the lab is ready for the day. You're already ahead of the game if you have the first-in, last-out mentality. Even just a few minutes of one-on-one time with somebody gives you that edge and the opportunity to get to know someone. You don't need to be best friends with everybody, but you never know who will be looking to help fill a job in the field one day.

I am a friendly, considerate, patient person who gets along with almost everybody. However, a woman in my echo class had a strong personality, was a know-it-all, and was hard to get along with. Fortunately, she was in the lab while I was in lecture class and vice versa. During our lecture, one day, she came barging in, accusing people of not cleaning up after themselves in the lab. For some reason, it was semi-directed at my lab group, which I, of course, took offense to. We had a bit of a spat in the middle of the classroom. It was embarrassing and childish. As time passed, I discovered she was intelligent and passionate about becoming an excellent tech. Just like, well, me. Gradually, we mended fences through mutual respect and the understanding that we were both there to excel in the classroom and lab and become successful in the field. A little less than a year after graduation, the phone rang, and she told me the lab she was working in was looking for a tech and asked if I might be interested. I also have had opportunities to recommend fellow students with whom I not only felt were qualified but with whom I built a solid relationship.

**Benefits of Networking**

1. **Opportunity Discovery**: Many job opportunities have yet to be advertised. Networking can help you access the hidden job market and learn about openings through referrals and recommendations.

2. **Insight and Advice**: Networking provides access to industry experts and mentors who can offer valuable insights, guidance, and advice on navigating your career path.

3. **Skill Development**: Engaging with a diverse network allows you to gain new perspectives and skills, enhancing your professional growth and adaptability.

4. **Support System**: A strong network can offer moral support, encouragement, and practical help during challenging times or career transitions.

**Build Your Network:**

1. **Start With Who You Know**: Connect with people you already know, such as classmates, teachers, and lab assistants. They can introduce you to others in your field or offer valuable advice.

2. **Attend Industry Events**: Conferences, workshops, and seminars are excellent places to meet professionals in your field.

3. **Join Professional Organizations**: Joining industry associations or professional groups can provide access to a network of like-minded individuals and opportunities for professional development.

4. **Be Genuine**: Authenticity is key. Approach networking with a genuine interest in others rather than a transactional mindset. Building authentic relationships requires listening, empathy, and mutual respect.

5. **Ask Questions**: Show interest in the people you meet by asking about their work, experiences, and perspectives. This not only helps you learn but also makes the conversation more engaging.

6. **Follow-up**: After meeting someone, send a follow-up message to express your appreciation for the conversation and suggest a way to stay in touch. This helps solidify the connection and keeps the dialogue going.

7. **Offer Value**: Networking is a two-way street. Look for ways to assist others in your network by providing information, making introductions, or offering support. This builds goodwill and strengthens relationships.

You don't have to go it alone. Once you build a multi-beneficial two-way street with your colleagues, you commit to helping each other. Late one afternoon, shortly after I was officially on the clock at the hospital, I ran into some difficulty during a routine lower extremity duplex exam. The only other tech still there would be leaving for the day shortly. After sweating through my scrubs, I gave her a call. She was one of the techs I had been shadowing frequently during my externship. She had one foot out the door and headed for home, but without hesitation, she made her way back through the long halls of the hospital to give me a hand. She knew I would do the same for her in a heartbeat. I saw many examples of this during my externship and many more once I was in the field. As an ultrasound tech, you can feel isolated and alone. It's just you, the machine, and the patient. Scanning and obtaining all the right images is not a team sport. Building a dynamic network that you can call upon and who can call on you when needed is critical.

After my externship, I was hired at the hospital. I know the "fill the gel bottles" mentality was crucial to this. It certainly was not because of my scanning skills. I was able to get hired without an actual interview, which would usually include demonstrating scanning prowess and or a written or verbal exam of skills and knowledge. I could bypass this part because I had already gained the techs' and department's respect and confidence.

# PATIENTS AND PATIENCE

"ALL WE NEED IS JUST
A LITTLE PATIENCE."
-GUNS AND ROSES

"All we need is just a little patience." A beautiful lyric by one of the greatest rock bands of all time, Guns and Roses, says it all. If you want to get familiar with this song, you can search it up and have it available in times of need. It may just become an anthem for you. To be a successful ultrasound tech, you will have to work with patients; with that, you'll need an endless supply of patience.

A fantastic instructor once told the story of the "Walker." This is not a zombie story, but it might feel like one when it inevitably happens to you. This situation will happen consistently and without warning. You're having a busy day. The schedule is packed, and you must catch up due to challenging studies, late patients, and poor front-office scheduling. The front-office staff needs help understanding how long it takes to do a lower extremity arterial study and a carotid study on one patient. You've told them you need at least 30 minutes per study, but they are scheduling patients 15 minutes apart. Thankfully, you see the next patient is a lower extremity venous study so that you can catch up. Here comes the "Walker." I can still see my instructor demonstrating this, which was humorous then, but not so much when you have not had lunch, and the office will close soon.

You go to the waiting room to get the patient. The patient is elderly, overweight, and uses a walker. You can whip them right into the treatment room with a wheelchair. Not with a walker. The walk from the waiting room to the treatment room, which usually takes about a minute, now becomes what feels like an hour. This is the time to take a deep breath and call forth those patience reserves. Although it feels like they will never get to the treatment room, they do, and it often turns out that they are the sweetest patients and the most effortless study of the day.

Indeed, one of the most fascinating and challenging aspects of patient care is dealing with diverse personalities. You never know what type of personality may walk through your facility's doors or what kind of character you may encounter when you enter a patient's room. Each patient is different, which can significantly impact how they perceive and respond to medical treatment. As healthcare professionals, we must provide the best care we can in any situation. This is going to take practice. We can't control what type of patients we may encounter daily, but one thing we can control is what we bring into the room. This is crucial when interacting with patients, co-workers, and management. It may help if you take a pocket full of patience and a scoop of empathy to work daily.

Empathy may be the cornerstone of patient care. Practicing active listening is essential to effectively connecting with patients of different personalities. Pay close attention to verbal and nonverbal cues. These cues can help you tailor your approach to diverse characters.

Your ability to adjust your communication style can significantly enhance patient satisfaction and compliance. Establishing a positive rapport with patients is vital to successful interactions. Finding a bit of common ground or shared interests goes a long way in helping the patient feel comfortable. Your confidence and established expertise will help alleviate anxiety and foster cooperation, leading to a productive interaction.

Here are some of the personality types you may encounter:

(Sweet, Angry, Helpless, Distracted, The Fidgeter, Rude, Mean, Talkative, Silent, Sad, Scared, Stressed, Flirtatious, Inappropriate, Unconscious, Mental Illness).

I'm here to tell you it doesn't matter what personality you encounter; you must be yourself. If you consistently bring patience, compassion, empathy, respect, and confidence into the room, you will set yourself up for success no matter which personality you meet. Every patient is unique, with preferences and needs. By approaching each patient with an open mind, patience, and empathy, you can provide exceptional patient-centered care that respects the diversity of the human experience.

# EXTERNSHIP

"BE SO GOOD; THEY CAN'T IGNORE YOU."
-STEVE MARTIN

This is it. You're finally ready for your externship. Congratulations! You are armed with your questionable sonography skills and a vague understanding of what actual pathology looks like. Although your school has placed you in a desirable location close to your home, the clinic or hospital may still want to meet you first. Oh boy, you know what that means? Interview. That's right; this gig is not a lock. If the lab or hospital agrees to let you hang around for a few months, the manager may want to meet you first. What will you wear? What will they ask you? What should you do? You can relax. You've made it this far. This is just another step on your path. If you were going to interview at a bank, would you wear scrubs? No, of course not. Should you wear a suit or dress to an interview at a medical clinic? Maybe not. Should you wear your cheap, worn-out school scrubs? Not the best idea. A nice pair of scrubs or a casual outfit that shows you are a professional may do the trick. As far as what they may ask, your guess is as good as mine. Just be prepared and be yourself.

I know what you're thinking. Ultrasound Techs are relaxed, patient, and understanding, just like my fellow students and that excellent physics teacher. Wrong! In the field, the life of the ultrasound tech is usually fast-paced and often involves juggling many tasks at once. Teaching you is generally a low priority, and frequently, the tech assigned to you may feel saddled by the curious, wide-eyed student ready to jump into action. Think about this for a minute. It's your job to learn, but not their job to teach. Here's your challenge.

Remember that young hot ultrasound tech you saw on that episode of Gray's Anatomy? That's not you or me or anyone. Medical dramas may do a great job of making ultrasound look like an intense yet glamorous affair. Unfortunately, the reality can be much different. You may start the day put together, calm, cool, and collected, but by the time you've got lost for the tenth time trying to navigate the maze of hallways in a hospital and pretending you know exactly where you're going, you'll probably be pretty rattled. Don't worry; no one will expect you to get it right the first time, but you must figure things out and do it quickly. About that nice new pair of freshly ironed scrubs, don’t get used to them.

One of the best tips I received was from a professor in school who said, "Always keep a fresh pair of scrubs in your car." If the hospital or clinic provides them, don't worry; you can always grab a fresh pair; if not, keep a clean pair in the trunk of your car. If it's not the bodily fluids that get splashed on you one day, it will be ketchup, mustard, or that cold cranberry juice you've been craving for the last two hours.

Don't get me wrong; it's not all bodily fluids, dead-end hallways, and overworked techs. One of the best aspects of being in the field is the camaraderie among fellow techs. You'll form bonds with like-minded individuals with whom you can swap funny stories and, most importantly, learn from. The externship is also the first and best place for you to seek a job opportunity. The biggest catch-22 of this career is that there are many job opportunities for ultrasound techs who have the one thing you still need to gain: experience. This is your first and sometimes only opportunity to show the people in a position to hire you that you can do this. The key is to make not just a good but an outstanding impression. At the end of your externship, you want the department to think about how they will get the job done when you're not there anymore. It all starts with "filling the gel bottles." The funny thing about doing an ultrasound is that it doesn't matter how fancy your machine is, the body habitus of your patient, or even knowing the protocol; you need GEL to do an ultrasound study.

Imagine you're asked to take the machine to a patient's room and get set up for an Echo study, and the tech says he may let you acquire a few images at the end. The study is on the other side of the hospital from your department. You enter the room and let the patient know why you are there. You move all the furniture necessary to squeeze your machine in. The towels are positioned, and you raise the bed to the perfect height. The tech walks in just as you finish putting in all the patient information. He's in a good mood and impressed by your setup. He gets in position to do the study and asks, "Where's the gel? You break into a sweat. His look quickly changes as he stares at you with eyes, saying, "Don't tell me you forgot the gel." This story can go another way as well. You hand him the gel bottle. It's empty, and the bottle makes that farting noise as he tries to squeeze out the last dregs of cold gel. In either case, you will not acquire any images today, nor may you be first in line for that per diem job opening up in the last week of your externship.

Excelling in an externship is not just a matter of personal achievement but a gateway to future professional success. The skills, experiences, and connections gained during training can significantly impact your career trajectory. In this unique learning environment, you can apply classroom knowledge to real-world scenarios, cultivate valuable industry relationships, and prove your capabilities to potential employers. The importance of performing well at an externship extends beyond the immediate role, as it lays the foundation for a solid professional reputation and opens doors to new opportunities. By embracing the challenges, seeking growth, and consistently delivering exceptional results, you can position yourself for a future marked by continuous advancement and meaningful contributions.

## THE BEGINNING

"ALTHOUGH NO ONE CAN GO BACK AND MAKE A BRAND-NEW START, ANYONE CAN START FROM NOW AND MAKE A BRAND-NEW ENDING."
-CARL BARD

Now is your chance to leap into the great unknown. Does that sound scary? Are you still wondering where this leap may take you? I can tell you this: You'll never find out if you don't jump. In most cases, this leap will lead you to a better place where all your dreams will come true. Too much? Maybe not all your dreams, but at least some of them. This leap can and will open doors and lead you down hallways you never expected.

During my last month of externship, a door opened. The Lead Tech with whom I developed a strong working relationship gave me an opportunity. She informed me that a Vascular clinic in the area needed a tech ASAP. There would be no time for an interview or training; the gig would be mine if I could pull it off. I had only scanned a handful of real-life patients. I leapt. I had to meet the tech at the clinic the next day. She had gone once or twice before, so she would introduce me and show me around. On the way there the next day, I was excited, but mostly, I felt fear and anxiety.

This vascular clinic was the real deal. There was a Vascular Surgeon and an Interventional Radiologist who wanted answers and wanted them fast. The clinic was not an imaging center where a patient comes in and gets scanned, and the scan is read sometime in the future. This clinic was the end of the road. The intervention was going to be done or not going to be done partially and sometimes primarily on the study I would perform. There were just a few studies the first afternoon, and the tech who referred me did most of the scanning. I was to return by myself the next day. The excitement was gone this time on the way there, and all that remained was an almost crippling feeling of fear and anxiety, but I went anyway. I dove in, doing studies I had some knowledge of and some I needed to gain a fundamental understanding of. I had to fake it until I could make it. It could have gone better. I remember leaving that first day drenched in sweat, dry mouth, nauseous, and doubtful. This was not my first job, and being an ultrasound tech was career number three or so for me. Yet, still, I was overwhelmed. I am not a stress eater, but I remember sitting down and eating a whole pizza that afternoon.

I'm sure they were on to my inexperience, but I had a good attitude, and luckily, I was all they had for the moment. I quickly incorporated all the ideas mentioned in this guide. I learned quickly, and they were patient. At least the nurses and front office were patient. The doctors were semi-tolerant. The doctors often looked over my shoulder to get the information they sought. Stressful? Yes, but knowing what the doctor is looking for is helpful. The fear and anxiety faded slowly, and a warm feeling of accomplishment remained. The reward of being a critical part of a team that directly impacts the patients they treat was nice. By the way, I still work at this clinic a few days a month. I have also gone on to help one of the doctors develop and grow a successful private practice.

Often, I reflect on the leap I had taken into the unknown. I embraced the fear and discomfort, navigated the challenges, and emerged better on the other side. Starting a new career requires courage through self-discovery, growth, and transformation. My journey had begun. The door opened, and I leaped. I suggest you dive in head first as well when the time comes. You have the tools needed to succeed. The time you put into your ultrasound skills and knowledge, the relationship building, and the never-ending striving for self-growth will be crucial to your success. Good Luck, you got this.

# ABOUT THE AUTHOR

Ronald Douglas Eustis holds a bachelor's degree from the University of California at Santa Barbara and an associate's degree from the West Coast Ultrasound Institute. He is a registered vascular tech, a registered diagnostic cardiac sonographer, and a certified personal trainer. He brings a rich tapestry of experiences to his writing, weaving tales that resonate with authenticity and depth. With a background in health, fitness, and the magical world of ultrasound, he has honed his craft through a blend of passion and dedication. Ronald enjoys spending time with his family, who continually inspire his creative journey.

# ACKNOWLEDGMENTS

I am deeply grateful to those who have inspired me and the creation of this book. I want to thank my teachers at West Coast Ultrasound and my colleagues Lorena, Denise, Kenia, Laura, and Vibol, who helped me weave through when I needed it the most. I also want to thank Dr Ali Golshan, a mentor and friend, for his unwavering support, patience, and knowledge and my friends and family for supporting me every day.

www.ingramcontent.com/pod-product-compliance
Lightning Source LLC
LaVergne TN
LVHW050346160826
845677LV00014B/3809

* 9 7 9 8 8 9 5 6 9 2 9 5 0 *